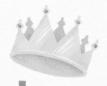

# Empowered Girls

## ACTIVITIES AND AFFIRMATIONS FOR EMPOWERING STRONG, CONFIDENT GIRLS

Allison Kimmey

**ILLUSTRATIONS BY CAIT BRENNAN**

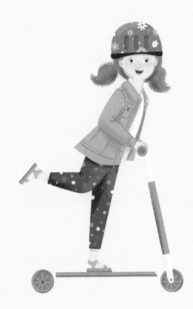

ROCKRIDGE PRESS

D1410873

*To my daughter, Cambelle, and my son, Graham,
for always pushing me to be the best woman I can be.*

For general information on our other products and services or to obtain technical support, please contact our Customer Care Department within the U.S. at (866) 744-2665, or outside the U.S. at (510) 253-0500.

Rockridge Press publishes its books in a variety of electronic and print formats. Some content that appears in print may not be available in electronic books, and vice versa.

Interior and Cover Designer: Amanda Kirk
Photo Art Director/Art Manager: Sue Bischofberger
Editor: Elizabeth Baird
Production Editor: Rachel Taenzler
Illustrations © 2021 Cait Brennan
Author photo courtesy of Winship Photography

ISBN: Print 978-1-64876-670-1
R0

# This Book Belongs To:

~~~~~~~~~~~~~~~~~~~~~~~~~~~~~~~~~~~~~~

# Contents

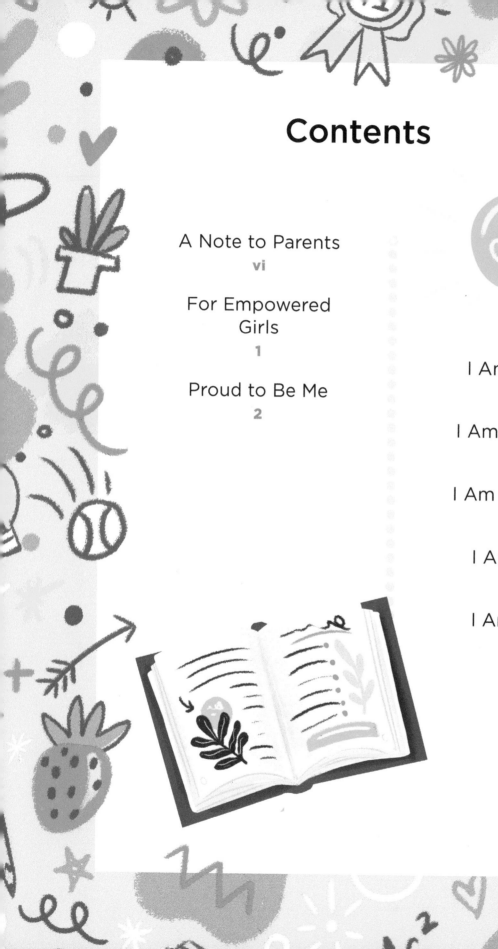

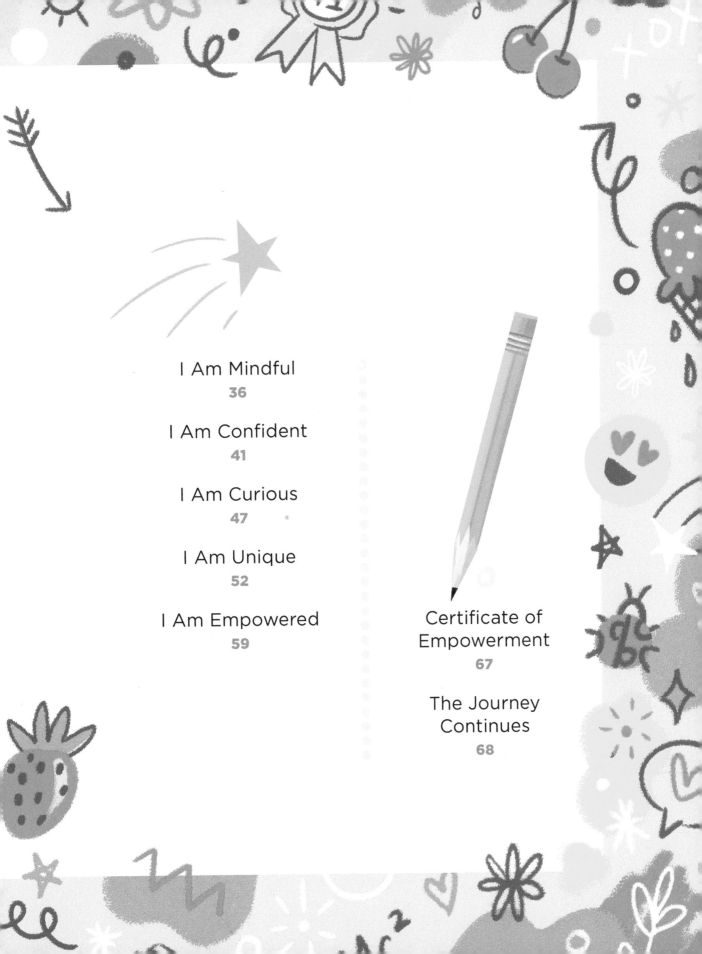

# A Note to Parents

It's important now more than ever for young girls to feel confident, secure, and empowered in their day-to-day lives. That's where this book comes in. Inside, your daughter will find empowerment-building activities to help her learn how incredibly special and valuable she is.

Encourage your daughter to make this book her own. There are plenty of pages for her to color however she likes, and spaces for her to fill with her thoughts and drawings. The activities can be done in any order. When your daughter needs a little extra help being calm, for example, she can check out the mindful chapter for suggestions. Or, if she is feeling creative, there are fun ideas to keep her inner artist busy.

Together, we can help your girl be the best she can be!

# For Empowered Girls

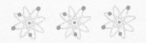

Hello, readers! My name is Allison Kimmey, but you can call me Miss Allie. My job is to help girls of all ages learn how to love themselves. no matter who they are.

I have a young daughter named Cambelle. She is the reason I wanted to write this book. When I was a girl, I didn't have a book like this to read. It sure would have helped me feel empowered and secure! I decided to put together fun activities for girls like you and Cambelle to help you feel confident in who you are. You are amazing! This book will help you see all the reasons why.

## What Does Empowerment Mean?

What is empowerment? It's a big word with a very import-ant meaning. When you are empowered, you are strong and confident in yourself. Being an empowered girl means that you are smart, beautiful, creative, kind, bold, mindful, confident, curious, and unique—and you *know* it.

Each section in this book begins with an affirmation. Affirmations are positive things you say to yourself, like "I am smart." Then, the activities in the section will show you how you embody that quality. Every time you complete a section, you'll grow a little bit more empowered. At the end of the book, you will receive an official Certificate of Empowerment (page 67). Let's get started by getting to know YOU!

# AGE

## Name

# PROUD

I LIVE IN

BIRTHDAY

MY FAMILY

MY PETS

## MY FRIENDS

to be ME!

FAVORITES

SCHOOL SUBJECT

SONG

HOBBIES

MOVIE

SPORT

WHAT I HOPE TO LEARN
FROM THIS BOOK

COLOR

FOOD

_____

_____

_____

# · I AM ·
# SMART

**YOU ARE SMART!** I bet you like to learn new things every day. This is called having a growth mindset, because learning new things helps your brain grow. You will never stop learning, even when you are old. Remember that everybody is smart in different ways—including you. Smart girls know that even though they might not be able to do something right now, with hard work, and maybe a little help, they will get better at it.

A+

EMPOWERED
GiRLS
Activities and Affirmations for
Empowering Strong, Confident Girls

Ages
6-9

# The Talent Tree

Everyone is good at something, and I know that you are good at LOTS of things! Maybe you're great at math, drawing pictures, or making up silly new songs. Maybe you give the best advice. Fill your talent tree with all the things you know you're great at—in school, at home, and with your friends, too. Hint: Think of some things you love doing.

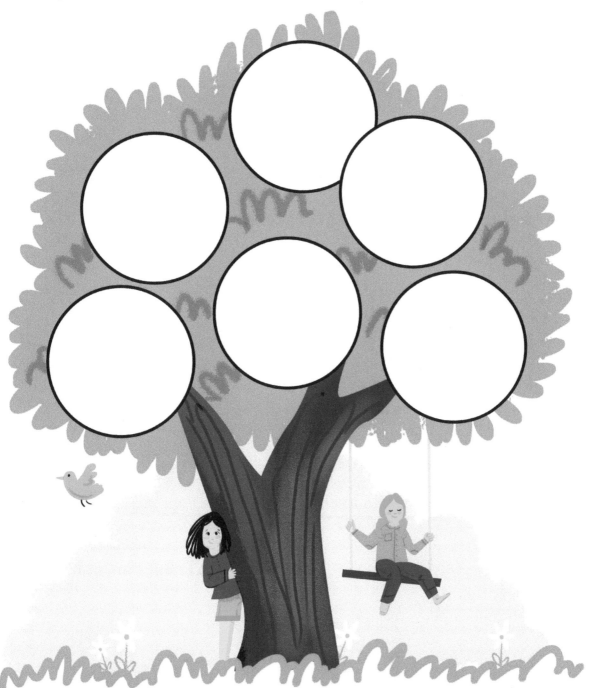

# The Power of YET

Sometimes you might not be great at something the first time you try it. Not being able to do something yet doesn't mean you can't be great at it someday. This is what we call the "Power of Yet." It means that if you keep trying, you WILL learn to do it in your very own way. Instead of saying, "I can't do that," and giving up, say, "I can't do that—YET!" and keep trying!

 Fill in the blanks below with some new and fun things you want to learn.

I'm not good at ................................................................

........................................**YET**, but if I work hard, I will be!

I can't ................................................................

........................................**YET**, but with practice, I'll be

able to.

I don't know how to ................................................................

........................................**YET**, but I know it takes

time, and I will figure it out soon!

I haven't been able to ................................................................

........................................**YET**, but if I ask

for help, I know I will succeed!

I'm not good at ................................................................

........................................**YET**,

but my abilities grow and change every day.

I can't ................................................................

........................................**YET**, but I am still

a smart girl!

# It's Okay to Ask for Help

No matter how smart you are, sometimes you need a little help. Asking for help can feel hard, because you don't want others to think you can't do something. Smart girls know that one of the best ways to get better at something is to ask someone who already does it well.

**These are some things that I might need help with:**

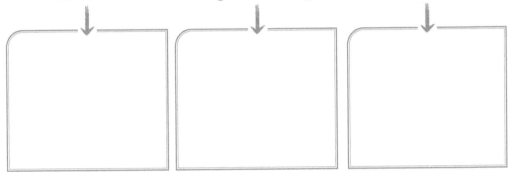

**These are some people I can ask for help when I need it:**

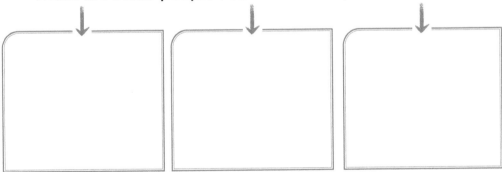

**These are some things that I can help other people with:**

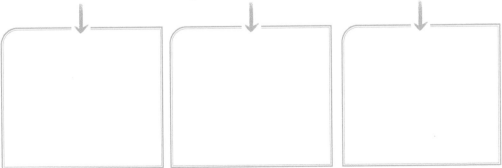

# Accomplishments Time Line ☑

You've already done *a lot* of things that prove how smart you are. Maybe you finished your first chapter book, answered a question correctly in class, or helped a younger sibling with a problem. Use the time line on this page to remind yourself of all that you have already accomplished. You can do anything you set your mind to. Just look at all you've done!

## My Time Line

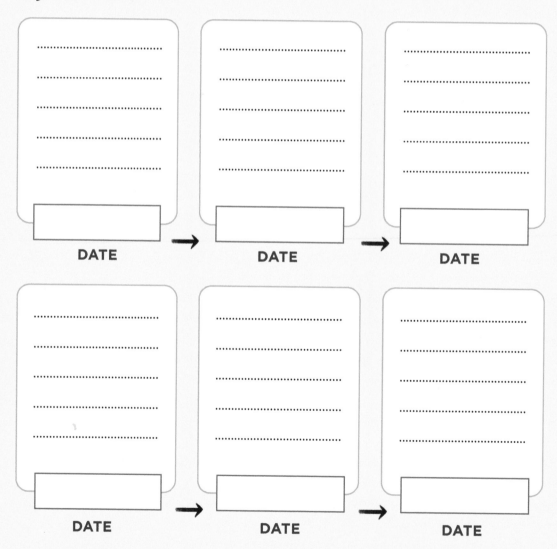

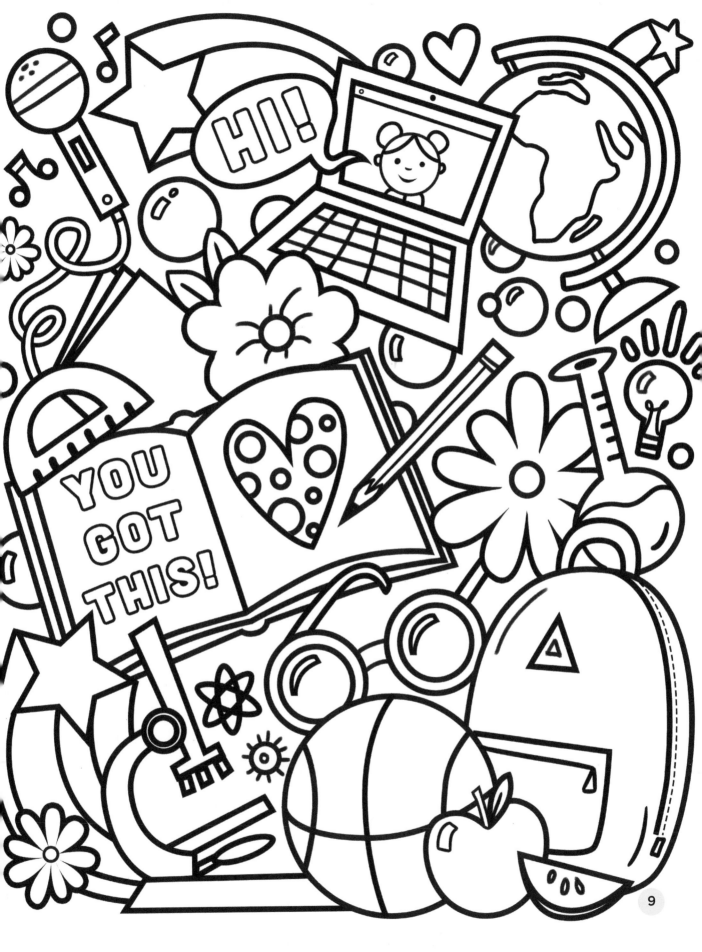

# I AM CREATIVE

**YOU ARE CREATIVE!** Your imagination is one of the most fun things about you. It allows you to explore faraway places and pretend to be things and people you're not. Do you know how else you can use your creativity? By imagining yourself with ALL of your best qualities—the most empowered you there could ever be. It's also helpful to imagine yourself doing hard things before you do them. It will help your confidence grow!

EMPOWERED GiRLS

Activities and Affirmations for Empowering Strong, Confident Girls

# Super Girl!

Did you know you already have superpowers? The power to be creative is one of them. Have fun with your imagination right now. Imagine yourself as a superhero. What superpowers would you love to have, and why? Would you be invisible? Able to fly? How would you use your powers to help the world?

*If I were a Super Girl, my superpower would be:*

*If I had superpowers, the first thing I would do is:*

*The most awesome superpower I have in real life is:*

# Finish the Story

Creative writing is a wonderful way to express yourself.
No one else thinks quite like you, and that makes you
very special! Fill in the blanks to create your very own story.
Read it to a friend or family member.

_capten un_ **Saves the Day**
HERO'S NAME

_Lola_ was just a normal girl, until one day she
HERO'S NAME

_ran_ into a _Sp_ . All of a sudden, she
VERB, PAST TENSE        NOUN

was able to _invisu dl_. She decided she needed a superhero name,
SUPERPOWER

so she called herself _caten un_. She wore a _Ren_
SUPERHERO NAME        COLOR

cape and _green_ shoes. One day, there was a loud _uau_!
COLOR OR ADJECTIVE        TYPE OF SOUND

A _ham str_ had _Jupet_ into a _toolet_.
NOUN        VERB, PAST TENSE        NOUN

Her _school_ needed help! She gathered a couple of her other
NOUN

super girl friends, _addy_ and _gg_.
SUPER FRIEND        SUPER FRIEND

They all used their superpowers to _hug_,
SUPERPOWER

_fly_, and _inviso_.
SUPERPOWER        SUPERPOWER

**Together, they saved the day!**

# Turn a Mistake into Art

It can be really embarrassing to make mistakes, even though EVERYBODY makes them. The cool thing about mistakes is that you can use your creativity to turn them into something beautiful. Here's a fun activity that proves that, with just a little creativity, there is beauty in our mistakes.

Oops! Someone accidentally made some scribbles in these frames. What creative drawings can you make from them?

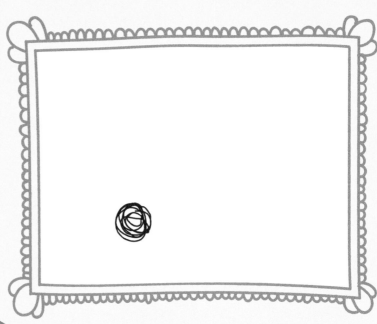

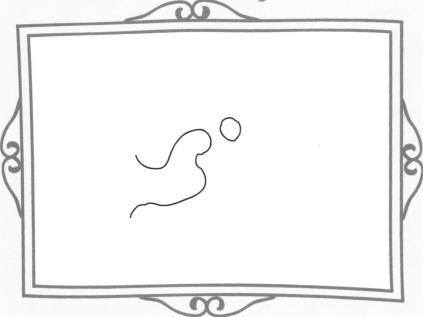

# Creative Girl Collage

A collage is a collection of different pictures or materials that you put together on a piece of paper. This one will tell a story about you. Your collage should be full of your favorite words, pictures, colors, or anything else that makes you smile.

**What You Need:**

**Scissors**
**Poster board**
**Glue**
**Other materials**
**of your choice:**
**magazine cutouts, photos,**
**ribbon, fabric, glitter**

1. Start by cutting out the words and pictures on this page, then cut out other fun pictures and letters from magazines.

2. Arrange the objects on the poster board.

3. When you're happy with how everything looks, glue down all the pieces. Add extra materials, like ribbon or glitter, if you want.

4. Hang your finished collage in your room.

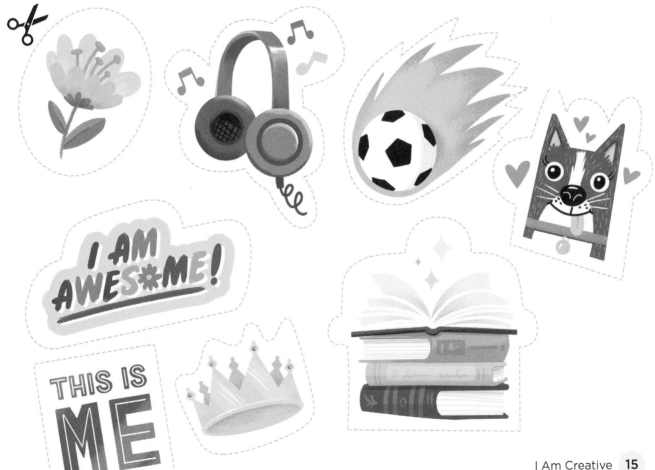

I AM AWES*ME!

THIS IS ME

# ·I AM·
# BEAUTIFUL

**YOU ARE BEAUTIFUL!** Can I tell you something, though? The way you look is not the most important part of being a beautiful person. Being beautiful also means having a kind heart and an open mind. It's easy to see other girls and compare how you look to how they look. But always remember that every person is beautiful in different ways. It's fun to celebrate and love what makes us different and beautiful—inside and out.

EMPOWERED
GiRLS

Activities and Affirmations for
Empowering Strong, Confident Girls

Ages
6-9

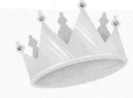

# Beautiful Me

Every single person is beautiful in their own way. In this activity, you're going to think about all the things that you love about YOU.

I love my

..................................

hair and

..................................

eyes.

I love how
my smile is

..................................

..................................

I love that I look like

..................................

..................................

I love that
I know how to

..................................

..................................

I love that
my skin is

..................................

..................................

I love that my body
can play

..................................

..................................

I love that my family
and friends say I am

..................................

and ..................................

# It's What's Inside That Matters

Have you ever heard of inner beauty? It is so much more important than what people see when they look at you. Some things that build your inner beauty are kindness, bravery, honesty, and being there for others. These things not only help you feel really great about yourself but also help others feel good.

Write things inside the figure that make your inner beauty really shine. Choose from the following words, or come up with your own.

Boldness

Compassion

Confidence

Honesty

Intelligence

Loyalty

Sense
of humor

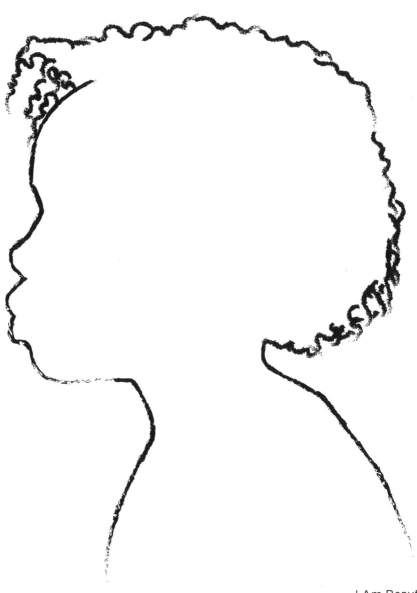

# Mirror, Mirror

It's time to be an artist! Grab some crayons or markers, find a mirror to look into, and get ready to draw a selfie (or self-portrait). Drawing yourself is a great way to admire how beautiful you really are. Keep in mind that you can draw what you see in the mirror, or you can use fun shapes and different colors to show how you see yourself or how you feel on the inside.

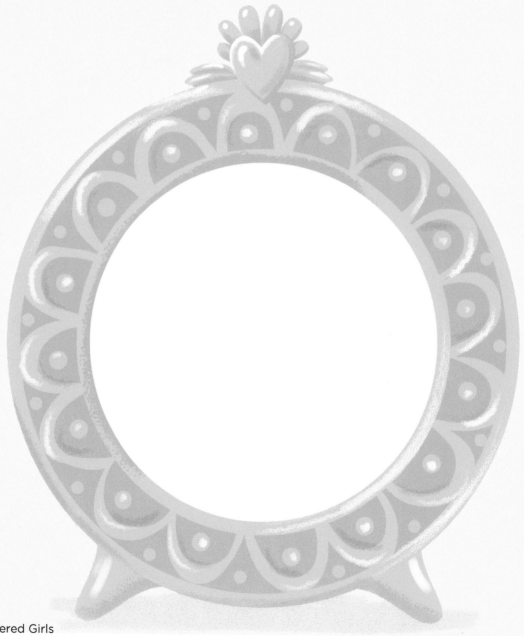

# My Beautiful Bestie

It's always wonderful to appreciate your own beauty, but it's also fun to admire someone else's. Isn't it crazy to know that there are almost eight billion people on the planet—and none of us look exactly the same? Use this page to celebrate the beauty of one of your besties. Draw them, then write down the things that make them such a great friend.

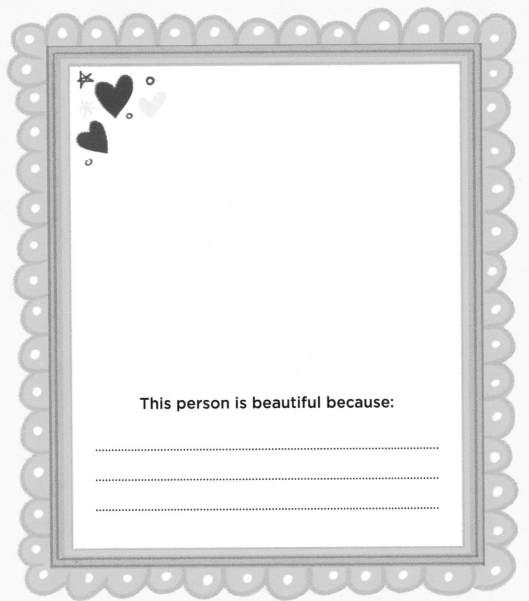

**This person is beautiful because:**

.................................................................................................

.................................................................................................

.................................................................................................

# · I AM ·
# KIND

**YOU ARE KIND.** I've always believed that being kind is one of the absolute best things you can be. Kind girls are compassionate, respectful, and helpful to others. There are so many ways to show your kindness with the words you say and the ways you help people, animals, and even the earth around you. The best part is that it always feels really good to know that you were the reason someone smiled today!

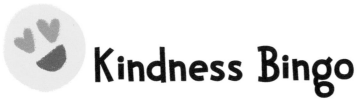

# Kindness Bingo

Let's make kindness fun with a game called "Random Acts of Kindness Bingo." Random acts of kindness are nice things you do for others or the planet without expecting anything in return. Look at the chart below. After you complete an act, put an X in its box. You win when you fill in a row across or down. It would be even more fun to fill the whole card. That would be a lot of kindness!

| Write a thank-you note. | Help someone before they ask. | Fill a bag of toys to donate. |
| --- | --- | --- |
| Recycle your trash. | Help clean up the classroom. | Give someone a compliment. |
| Volunteer at an animal shelter. | Bake a dessert for a neighbor. | Share your snack with a friend. |

# Be Kind to Yourself

Being kind to yourself is just as important as being kind to others. Here are some things you can do to show yourself some love and care.

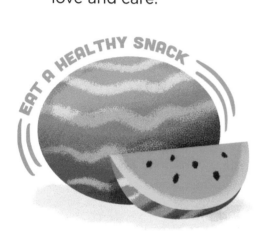

**EAT A HEALTHY SNACK**

**WATCH A FUNNY MOVIE**

**GET SOME EXERCISE**

**GIVE YOURSELF A COMPLIMENT**

**TAKE A DEEP BREATH**

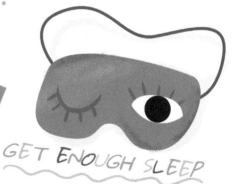

**Enjoy the Outdoors**

**ASK A GROWN-UP FOR HELP**

**VISIT A FRIEND**

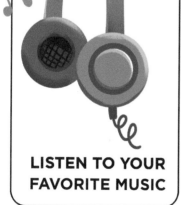

**LISTEN TO YOUR FAVORITE MUSIC**

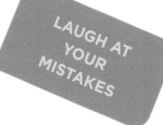

**LAUGH AT YOUR MISTAKES**

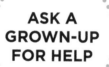

**GET ENOUGH SLEEP**

# Kindness Journal

Have you heard the phrase "pay it forward"? It means that when you are kind to others, they are often kind to someone else in return. People do kind things for us all the time. Can you think of a time when someone did something extra nice for you? Write about it here.

...................................................................................................

...................................................................................................

...................................................................................................

...................................................................................................

Think about how you could do something kind for someone else to "pay it forward." What would you do? Draw yourself doing it.

# A Sprinkle of Kindness

We've talked about many different ways you can brighten someone's day by being thoughtful. Now, it's your turn. Get ready to sprinkle this ice cream cone with kindness. On each sprinkle below, write a way you can be kind to others or yourself. Kindness is sweet, and so are you!

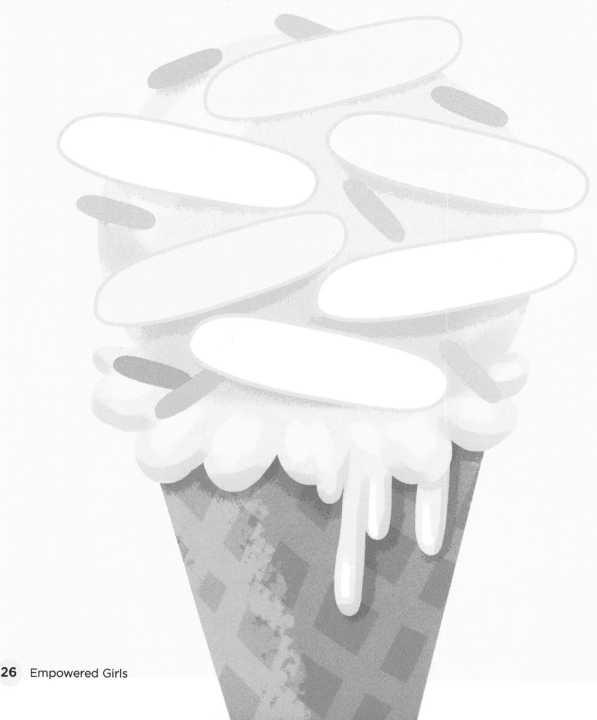

# Create a Card

Think about the people you are thankful for. Some of them do their jobs without hearing the words "thank you" very often. This is where you come in. Complete the card on this page, cut it out, then give it to someone special. Like who?  Some good ideas are: a parent or grandparent, a best friend, your teacher, a postal worker, a nurse, or a grocery clerk. Watch their face light up when they get their card. They will love it!

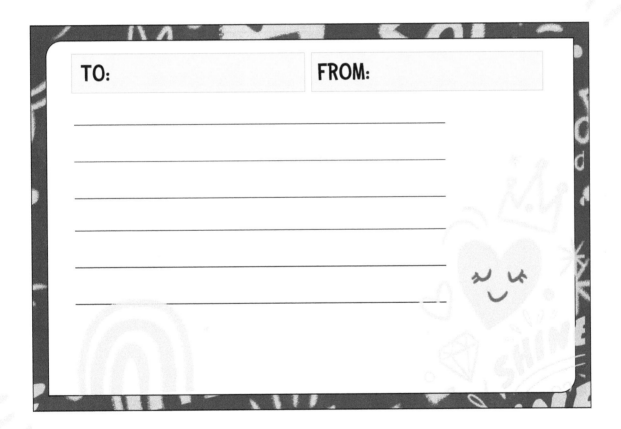

TO:                          FROM:

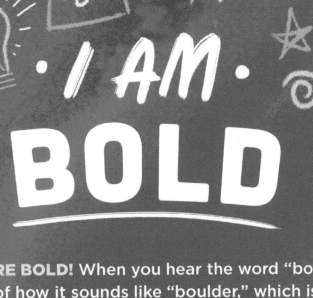

# · I AM ·
# BOLD

**YOU ARE BOLD!** When you hear the word "bold," think of how it sounds like "boulder," which is a big rock. Being bold is like being a boulder. It stays strong even when people push it. It's too big to hide and takes up a lot of space. You are bold when you take chances and don't worry about what someone else might think. A bold girl stands up for what is right, even when no one else will. Bold girls dream big and won't let anything get in their way!

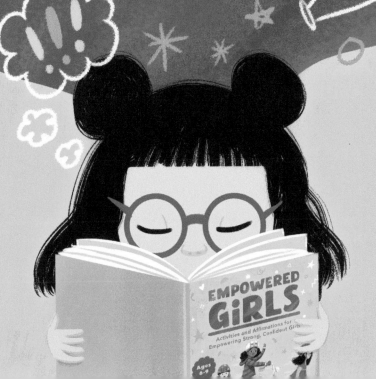

# Loud and Proud

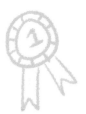

Here's a cheer for you to try. Just put your name into the blank, and say it out loud. *I am* ........................................ *and I couldn't be prouder. If you can't hear me, I'll yell a little louder!*

Now it's your turn. Complete the sentences below. They will help you figure out your boldest goals. Then, take this book with you to the mirror and read your sentences out loud. It might feel silly at first, but saying things out loud can actually help you believe them!

## My Bold Statements

**When I grow up, I will be a** ............................................
............................................................................**.**

**I am not afraid to** ......................................................
............................................................................**.**

**I love myself even if** ...................................................
............................................................................**.**

**I will always stand up for** ....................................**,**
**because it is the right thing to do.**

**Someday, I will have the courage to** ..........................
............................................................................**.**

**I am bold, because I** .....................................................
............................................................................**.**

# Draw Your Wildest Dreams

Do you ever think about what you want to be when you grow up? As a young girl, I wanted to be a singer. Then, in high school, I sang all by myself in front of a big audience. My dream came true. When you dream big dreams—and work on them when you are awake— you can make them happen. In the dream bubble, draw one of your wildest dreams that you would love to make come true.

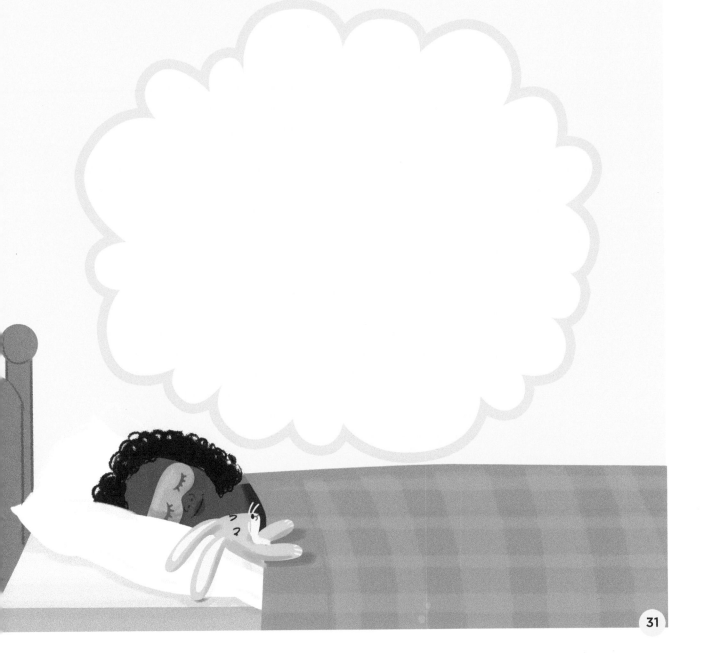

# Upstander or Bystander?

Bold girls are not afraid to do the right thing. Bullying is something you may see while you are with friends or at school. Bystanders may notice that someone is being bullied but don't say anything about it. Bold girls are upstanders. That means they don't just watch hurtful behavior. They do something about it. They stand up for the person being bullied and speak up. Take the pledge below and promise to always stand up for what is right.

## Anti-Bullying Pledge

I, ................................................. , agree to join together
**NAME**
with my peers to STOP bullying.

### I will **RESPECT** others by:

• including anyone who is left out

• encouraging others rather than putting them down

• choosing NOT to be a bully

### I will **HELP** others by:

• REFUSING to watch, laugh, or join in when someone is being bullied

• telling an adult when I see someone being teased or hurt

Signed by: ...............................................................

Date signed: ...............................................................

# Courageous Comic

Do you remember a time that you did something really brave?
Maybe you weren't even sure that you would be able to do it,
but you did. Use the comic boxes below to draw what happened.
Tell your story in the speech balloons. Your comic will show
everyone how you overcame the challenge to be a bold girl.

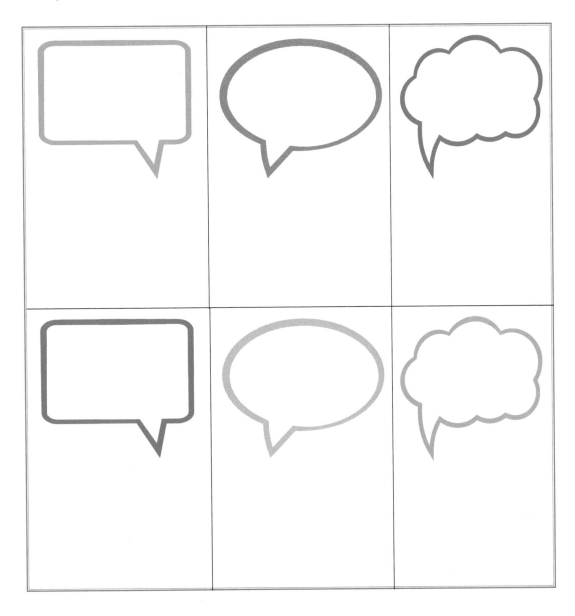

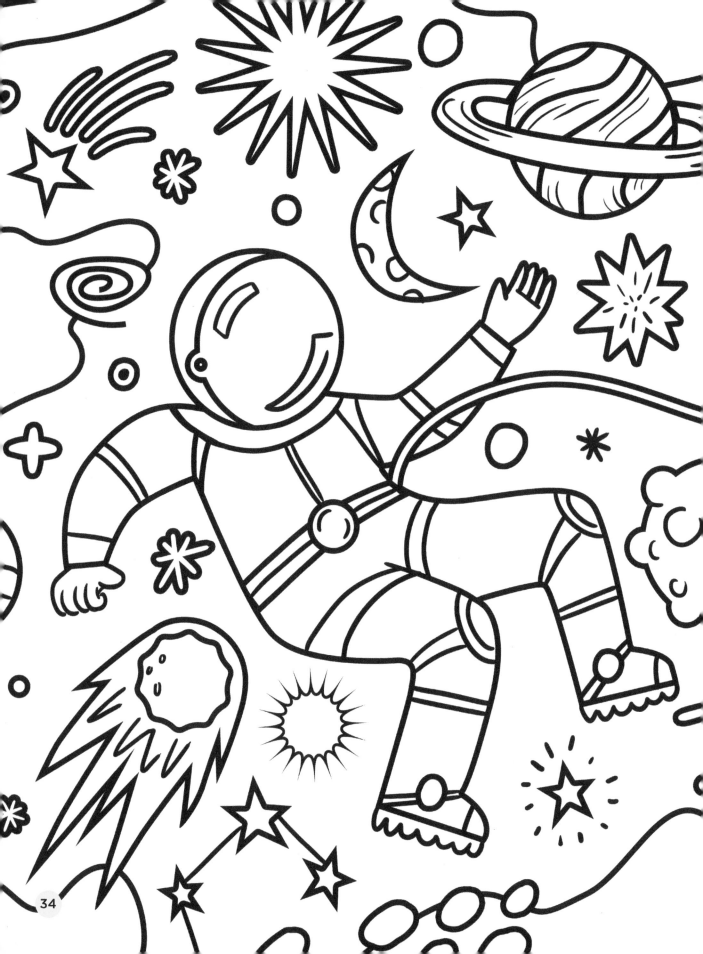

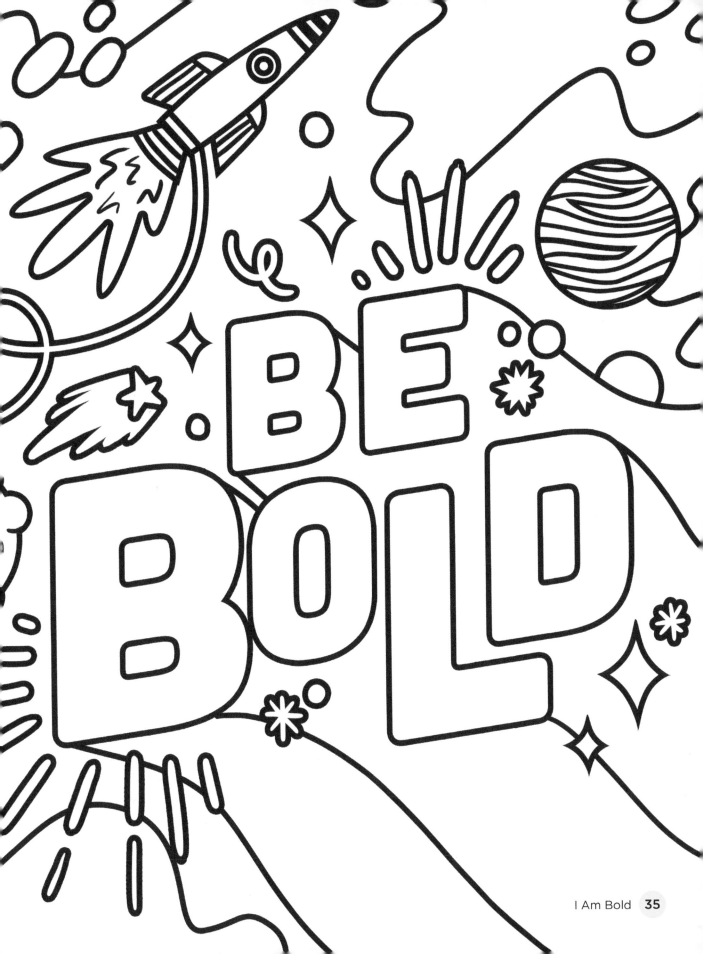

# · I AM · MINDFUL

**YOU ARE MINDFUL!** This means you make sure you notice all of your different emotions. It is very helpful to know what mood you are in and what made you feel that way. Mindful girls use a lot of different words to describe how they are feeling, such as happy, sad, nervous, or excited. They talk about those emotions with a grown-up. Mindful girls also have different tools to help control their emotions. Let's learn some now.

# Balloon Breath

Sometimes when you have big feelings, you might feel trapped or out of control. One of the best ways to remember that you are going to be okay is to practice slow breathing. This breathing activity is perfect for calming you down and helping you work through your feelings in a mindful way. Try this now and whenever you feel overwhelmed.

**Step 1:** Lie on your back on a rug, your bed, or a yoga mat. Close your eyes, if you like.

**Step 2:** Place your hands flat on your belly so your fingertips form a circle.

**Step 3:** Breathe in slowly through your nose for at least four seconds. Try to make your belly bigger, like a balloon filling up.

**Step 4:** Breathe out slowly. Let your belly get smaller, like the balloon is deflating.

**Step 5:** Repeat five times.

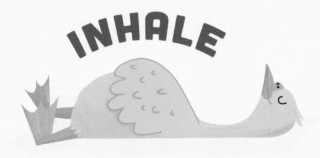

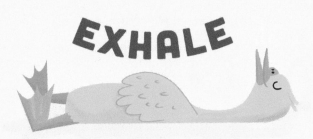

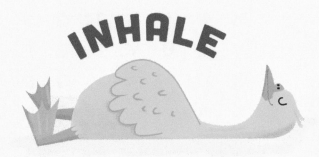

# Find the Feelings

We all experience lots of different emotions throughout our lives. Mindful girls know that they won't feel happy 100 percent of the time, and that's okay! Whatever you're feeling, it helps to talk about it with someone you trust. Find all the hidden emotions in this word search. You've likely felt all of these at some point!

```
D H X V N X X F G E J C S S L
X A C R E I Q B W P U W K D P
S P A X K B Y M Q C D U T H Q
O V L J Q O H R A J T C O I U
G J M I E M B A R R A S S E D
W O R R I E D R K E X Q R F J
L H P W C D I S G U S T E D N
E F S U R P R I S E D F M F B
B X A A Q P O G V S I L L Y H
F E C O Z G Y K P A M T R O A
G N U I A S P B S C A R E D P
W F I G T G S A D G W Z V C P
V L U Y E E F D E T K X D A Y
S D B J N Q D T I R E D X T T
L A F O S A N G R Y B U F X V
```

| | | | |
|---|---|---|---|
| Angry | Embarrassed | Sad | Surprised |
| Calm | Excited | Scared | Tired |
| Disgusted | Happy | Silly | Worried |

*See answers on page 69.*

# Up and Away

Big feelings can be hard to handle, especially if they have been hanging around for a little too long. You can help yourself feel better by letting go of some of those big thoughts. In the clouds on this page, write some thoughts that have been upsetting you. Maybe you fought with a friend, are missing someone, or are having a hard time at school. Imagine that the clouds are floating away with your thoughts. Do you feel better?

# The Mindful Minute

Getting in touch with your five senses is a fun way to be mindful. Do you know all five? They are sight, hearing, smell, taste, and touch. When you use your senses, you are focusing your brain on your eyes, ears, nose, mouth, and skin. This helps you concentrate on the present moment—not just your thoughts.

**Try taking a Mindful Minute. Close your eyes, sit quietly, and . . .**

**Smell**

Take a deep breath through your nose. Fill your lungs and think about what you smell.

---

**Hear**

Listen carefully to the sounds around you. What do you hear?

---

**Touch**

Use your fingertips to feel an item near you. Is it bumpy? Smooth? Soft?

---

**See**

Open your eyes and look at something near you. Think about its shape, size, and color.

---

**Taste**

Take a sip of water or juice and think about how it tastes and feels on your tongue.

# · I AM ·
# CONFIDENT

**YOU ARE CONFIDENT!** Being confident means that you are sure of your abilities, trust yourself, and know that you are more than enough just as you are. Confident girls try their best to be positive. They have the right words to say to others—and themselves—to make them feel accepted. The next activities will help you believe in yourself, walk tall, and show others that they can be confident, too.

EMPOWERED
GiRLS
Activities and Affirmations for
Empowering Strong, Confident Girls

Ages

# ⭐ Positive Pep Talk ⭐

You have thousands of thoughts every day. Unfortunately, sneaky negative thoughts can slip in from time to time. They even might make you start feeling bad about yourself. This activity will help you turn those negative thoughts into positive ones. Here are two columns of boxes. Write your negative thoughts in the boxes on the left. The ones on the right are for you to turn each negative into a positive. The first one is done for you.

| Negative Thoughts | Positive Thoughts |
| --- | --- |
| "I don't like that I am taller than everyone in my class." | "It is good to be this tall. I can help my shorter friends reach things!" |
| | |
| | |
| | |
| | |
| | |
| | |

# My Garden of Talents

Confident girls know what they're already great at. They also know that they can become great at anything, if they work hard enough. Write something you are *already* good at in the center of each pot that has a flower. In the pots that are just tiny seedlings, write talents you're going to work on over time. Keep watering these talents by practicing them. This will help your confidence grow!

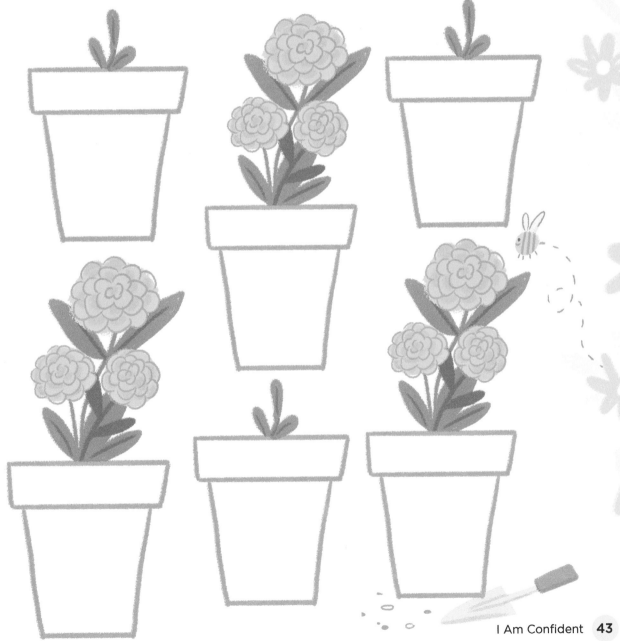

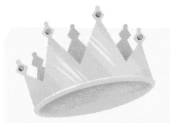

# Around the Table

Your confidence is contagious. That means that when you are confident in yourself, you can make others confident, too. You can also give them a little boost. Try this activity with a few friends or family members when having lunch or dinner at the table. Take turns telling each person around the table one thing you like about them. Get a head start and write down a few things that you really like about your favorite people below.

⭐ I like ............................... because .........................................
               **NAME**
.................................................................................................

⭐ I love when .................... is .........................................
                 **NAME**
.................................................................................................

⭐ My favorite thing about .................... is .....................
                       **NAME**
.................................................................................................

⭐ When .................... does ...........................................,
        **NAME**
it makes me happy.

⭐ .................... has the nicest ..................................
   **NAME**

⭐ I really like how .................... does .....................
               **NAME**
.................................................................................................

# Confidence Cutouts

When is the best time to be confident? All the time! Putting positive notes on your mirror or in your room can help you begin your day with a confident attitude. Color the notes below and add some that are unique to you. Cut them out and tape them to your mirror. Repeat the positive messages each morning.

# I AM
# CURIOUS

**YOU ARE CURIOUS!** What does this mean? You are always ready to learn new things. You ask lots of questions. You are a problem solver. Curious girls never stop finding answers. You might read a book, interview a person, or work to get something right. There are so many ways to be curious at home or at school. All of them help your brain and challenge you to grow.

EMPOWERED
GiRLS

Activities and Affirmations for
Empowering Strong, Confident Girls

Ages
6-9

# 5 Ws and 1 H

The best way to learn is by asking questions. Put on your thinking cap and interview someone to learn something from them. Pick a person and an interview topic. Here are some ideas: Ask about a favorite family recipe, find out why your teacher decided to become a teacher, or ask a grown-up about their childhood. During the interview, make sure that you get an answer to each of these questions: *What? Where? Why? Who? When? How?*

**I am interviewing:** ........................................

**I want to find out more about:** ....................

........................................................................

**What** ................................................................

........................................................................?

**Where** ...........................................................?

**Why** ...............................................................

........................................................................?

**Who** ...............................................................

........................................................................?

**When** .............................................................?

**How** ................................................................

........................................................................?

# The "I Will Try" Can

Are you curious to learn some new things? Maybe you want to learn how to do a backflip or try spaghetti squash. If you set your mind to it, you can do anything! Find a small, empty can, jar, or box. This is your "I Will Try" Can. Write things you want to try on small pieces of paper and put them in the container. Whenever you're feeling curious, grab an idea out of the can and try it.

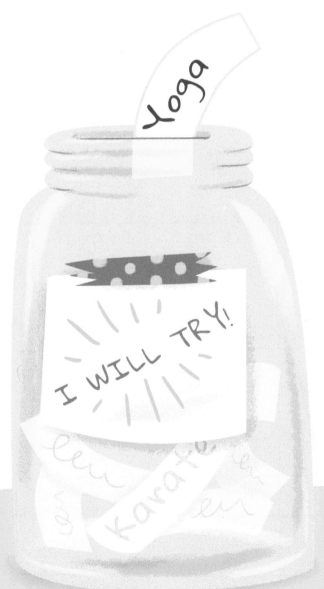

# Finding Adventure

Curious girls love adventures. After all, you never know what you might find or learn! One of the simplest adventures is going on a scavenger hunt in your neighborhood, at a park, or even around your house. You will need to stay curious during your hunt. Make sure you look in unexpected places to find all of the items, and write or draw what you found in the boxes below. How many did you find?

| FIND SOMETHING THAT . . . | | | |
|---|---|---|---|
| Is blue | Has four legs | Is flat | You can't live without |
| Beeps | Is wet | Is soft and fluffy | Is scratchy |
| Has wheels | Smells funny | Has buttons | Puts a smile on your face |
| Floats | Can hold things | Has more than five colors | Is taller than you |

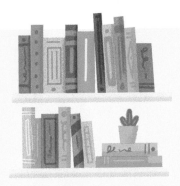

# Reading Race

Are you curious about the world around you? Read a book—or lots of them! Reading isn't just for homework. It's fun, too. Books can take you to faraway lands, teach you about your favorite animals, or help you learn about a very important person. Use this reading log to keep track of books you read. Put in the date you finished reading them as well as a short note about what you liked or learned about in each.

| READING LOG | | |
|---|---|---|
| Book | Date Completed | What I Liked or Learned About in This Book |
| | | |
| | | |
| | | |
| | | |
| | | |
| | | |
| | | |

# ·I AM·
# UNIQUE

**YOU ARE UNIQUE!** That means that there is only one you in the whole wide world. Unique girls know that their differences are what make them special. You might feel unsure about being unique, but we are going to celebrate exactly what makes you . . . YOU! Just think, if everyone was exactly the same, it would be a pretty boring world, right?

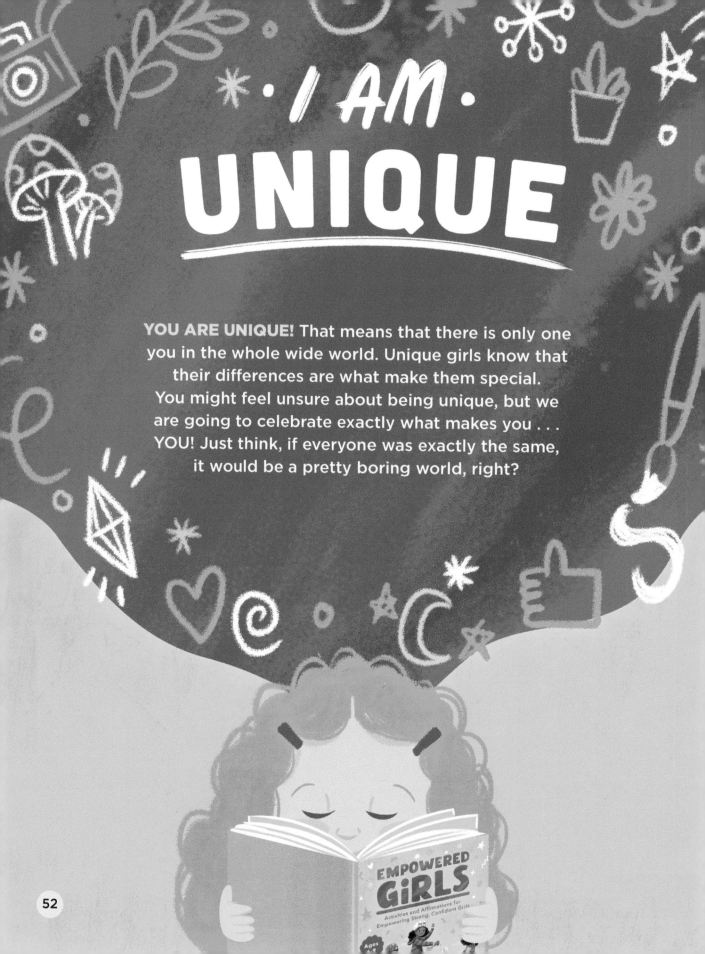

EMPOWERED
GiRLS
Activities and Affirmations for
Empowering Strong, Confident Girls

# Delightful Differences

It's important to celebrate and appreciate everyone's differences. Just because someone isn't the same as you doesn't mean you can't be friends. In fact, being different means you can learn things from each other. Pick a good friend or family member. Draw a picture of you and the other person in the boxes, then respond to the prompts.

| This is me: | This is ........................ : |
|---|---|
|  | NAME |

Ways ........................ and I are the same: ........................
NAME

........................

........................

Ways we are different: ........................

........................

........................

My favorite thing about ........................ is: ........................
NAME

........................

........................

# Fancy Fingerprints

Did you know that your fingerprints have a unique pattern that only belongs to you? Not only that, all of your fingerprints are different from each other. Want to find out what yours looks like? Try this fun activity!

**What You Need:**

**Pencil**
**Clear tape**

1. Color in the square below with a pencil until it's dark gray.

2. Firmly rub one fingertip onto the penciled square.

3. Press your fingertip onto the sticky side of a piece of tape.

4. Peel off the tape and stick it in one of the 10 spaces below.

5. Repeat with your other fingers. Now you can see the unique patterns of your fingerprints.

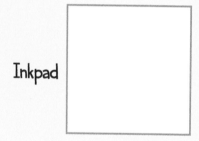

Inkpad

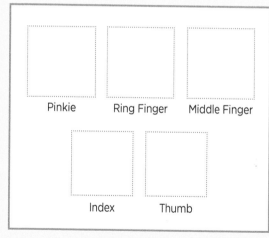

Left Hand

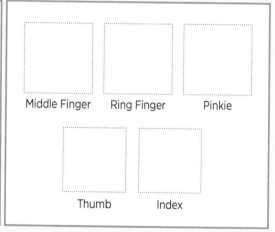

Right Hand

# Special Snowflakes

Like fingerprints, no two snowflakes are the same. This means
you actually have quite a lot in common with a snowflake.
Let's create one that is just as unique as you are!

**What You Need:**

**A square piece of paper**
**Scissors**

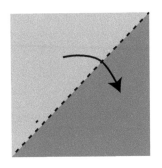

**1.** Fold the paper in
half diagonally
to make a
triangle.

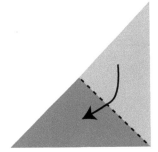

**2.** Fold in half once
more as shown
to create a
smaller triangle.

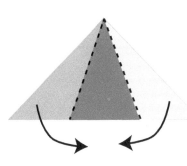

**3.** Fold this triangle
into thirds
by folding both
edges in.

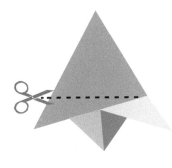

**4.** Your shape should
look like this.
Cut off the
points along the
dotted line to
make a triangle.

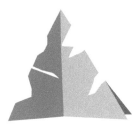

**5.** Carefully make
cutouts along
the edges to
create your
unique pattern.

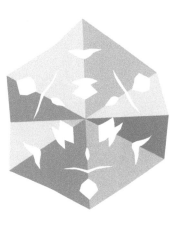

**6.** Unfold to see
your masterpiece.

# Fly Your Flag

Use your uniqueness to make your very own ME flag. Think about your unique talents, ideas, dreams, and goals. What makes you *you*? Why not also design one for a friend, brother, sister, or parent to celebrate what makes them special? Do you have some interests, goals, or dreams in common?

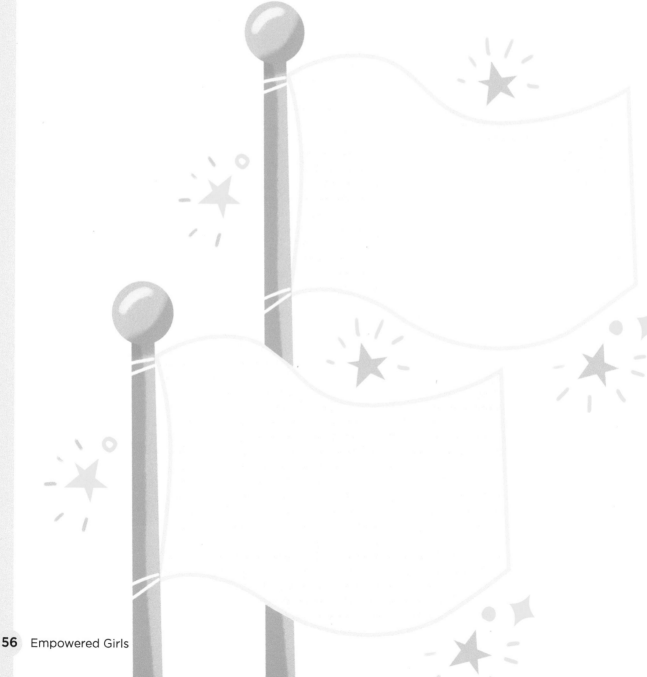

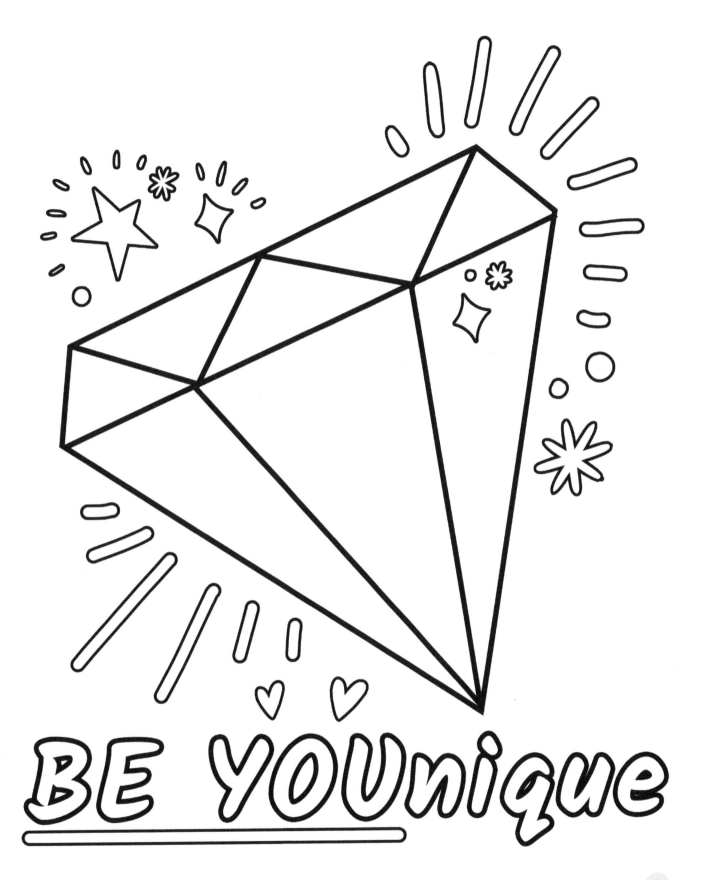

BE YOUnique

# ·I AM·
# EMPOWERED

**YOU ARE EMPOWERED!** By now, you've learned so much about yourself. You should know that you are perfect just the way you are. You love yourself, and you find the good in every person you meet. You aren't afraid to just be you. You focus on making good choices and feel confident to take on any challenge. You should feel proud, but there are a few more things I want you to know.

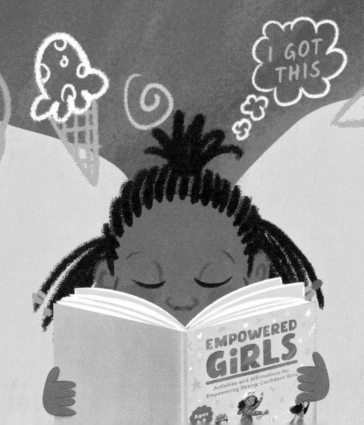

I GOT THIS

EMPOWERED GiRLS

Activities and Affirmations for Empowering Strong, Confident Girls

# Sometimes It's Okay to Say No

Empowered girls know when to say "yes" and when to say "no." It can be easy to want to say "yes" to everyone's needs or plans. But it's important that you know what people, activities, and situations make you feel uncomfortable. If there is something that you feel like you shouldn't be doing—or don't want to do—it's okay to politely pass. Here are some different ways to say "no."

**Just say "no":**
**"No, thanks."**

•

**Delay:**
**"No, not today. Maybe tomorrow."**

•

**Suggest a plan B:**
**"No, but how about**........................**?"**

•

**Be truthful:**
**"No, because**........................**."**

•

**Avoid:**
**"I can't. My mom needs me at home."**

•

**Leave the scene:**
**Say "no" and leave.**

# Power Pose

Standing tall makes you feel strong and like you can do anything. Your posture, or the way you stand, can improve how you feel about something difficult. Empowered girls use power poses to channel all their power and feel ready to do hard things. Practice this power pose the next time you are feeling a little nervous about trying something new.

1. Stand up straight, feet apart.
2. Roll your shoulders back and tilt your chin up.
3. Put your hands on your hips.
4. Hold this pose for two minutes while you think about how amazing and empowered you are!

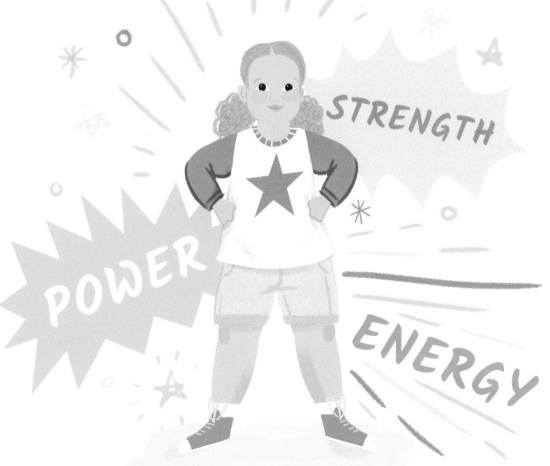

# Real Role Models

Empowered girls hang out with people who inspire them to do good things. There are many women—both past and present—who have made a big difference in the world. Learn the ways they were empowered to make their dreams come true. They can inspire YOU. Maybe you will be the inspiration for someone else one day!

Make a list of women who inspire you. Here are a few to get you started: **Rosa Parks, Helen Keller, Malala Yousafzai, Kamala Harris, Marie Curie, and Oprah Winfrey**.

**A woman who inspires me:** ......................................................

**She inspires me because:** ......................................................

......................................................................................

......................................................................................

......................................................................................

**A woman who inspires me:** ......................................................

**She inspires me because:** ......................................................

......................................................................................

......................................................................................

......................................................................................

**A woman who inspires me:** ......................................................

**She inspires me because:** ......................................................

......................................................................................

......................................................................................

......................................................................................

# Crown for a Queen

Empowered girls know that everyone should be treated with the same respect as royalty. Remind yourself of your value by making a beautiful crown. This origami crown is fit for a queen. Wear it proudly!

**What You Need:**

6 square pieces
  of paper, any color
Clear tape

Jewels or glitter
  (optional)
Glue (optional)

1. Fold a square of paper in half, from corner to corner.

2. Fold in half again as shown.

3. Unfold. Repeat these steps for all six pieces of paper.

4. Tuck one triangle's folded edge inside another as shown. Use a small piece of tape to keep it in place. Repeat until all six pieces are connected.

5. Tape together the two end pieces to complete the crown. Remove or add triangles as needed to fit your head.

6. Decorate with jewels and glitter, if you wish.

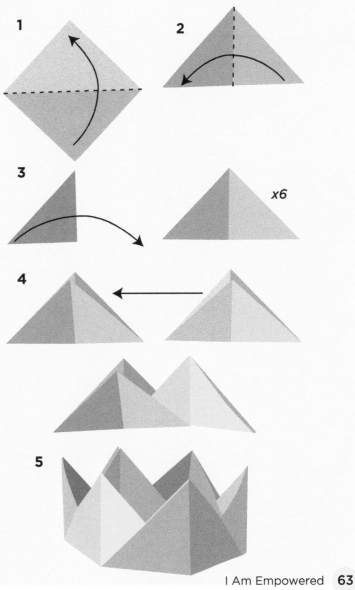

# Now It's Your Turn!

We learned a lot of affirmations together. Now it's time for you to write your own. Remember that an affirmation is just a positive sentence about yourself. Write your own affirmations in the bubbles. Once you've written them, make sure to say them out loud at least once a day. Try saying them while you are in your power pose (see page 61).

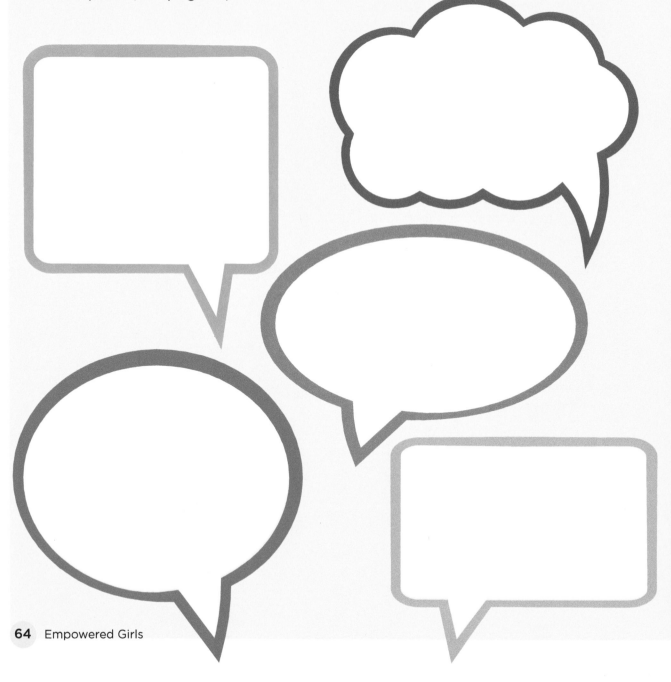

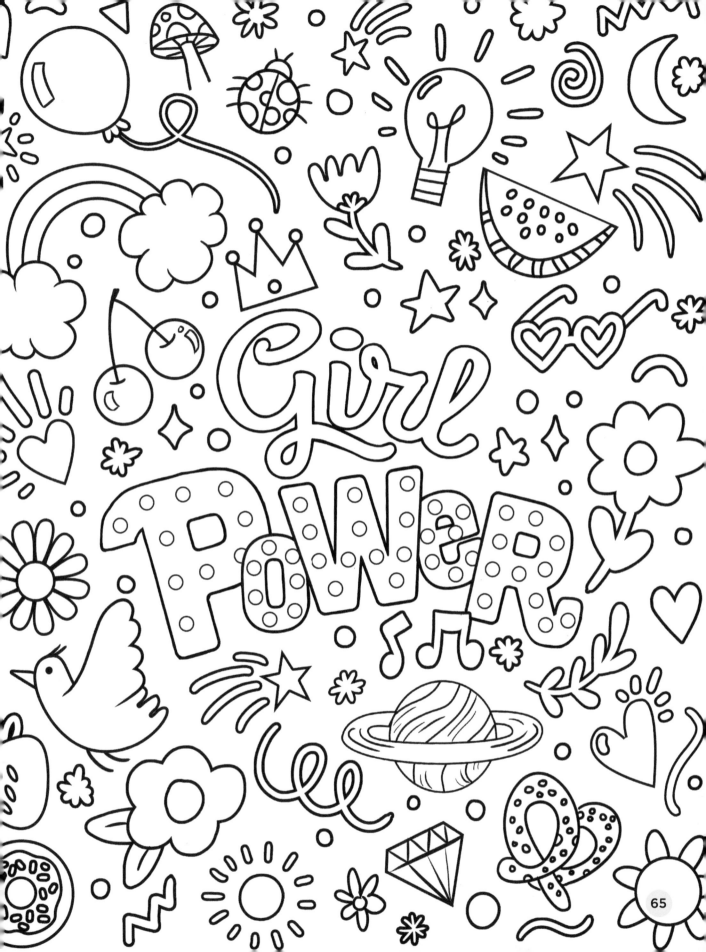

# CERTIFICATE OF EMPOWERMENT

## You Did It!

This certifies that .................................................... is empowered. She is smart, creative, beautiful, kind, bold, mindful, confident, curious, and unique. She will do her best to help others feel the same way.

Signature

....................................................

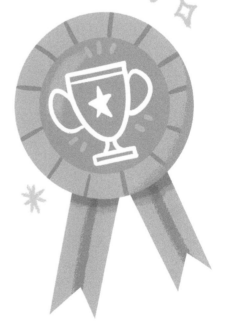

# The Journey Continues

It feels good to be empowered, right? Continue to grow your confidence with a website and books that celebrate empowered girls.

**A Mighty Girl: AMightyGirl.com**
Find books, movies, music, and more for smart and courageous girls here.

**Love Your Body** by Jessica Sanders
Everyone is beautiful in their own way. This book celebrates your amazing body and all it can do.

**Happy Confident Me Journal** by Nadim Saad and Annabel Rosenhead
This daily journal will help you discuss your feelings, focus on the positives, and inspire you to be the best person you can be.

**All of the Wonderful Things I Am: A Coloring Book for Girls**
by The Northern Star Printing Co.
Get creative while remembering that you are
smart, adventurous, imaginative, and confident.

**Good Night Stories for Rebel Girls: 100 Tales of Extraordinary Women**
by Elena Favilli and Francesca Cavallo
Be inspired by the adventures of 100 real
women of the past and present in this book
illustrated by 60 female artists
from around the world.

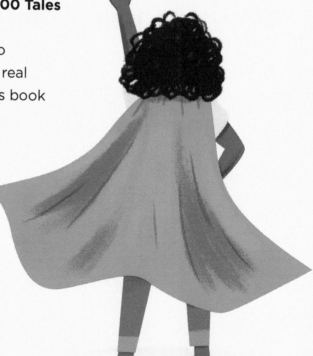

**You Are a Girl Who Totally Rocks!**
by Ashley Rice
Need a little reminder of how
incredible you are? This book is full
of inspirational notes that celebrate
your uniqueness.

# About the Author

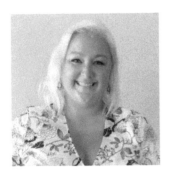

**Allison Kimmey** is a thirtysomething mom of two living along the sunny beaches of Florida with her high school sweetheart. Allie began sharing her self-love journey candidly on Instagram in 2016 and took the Internet by storm with her declaration that she found joy in a larger body. Allison uses her platform to help women of all shapes and sizes feel confident with her "Just Do You" mentality. Most important, she is dedicated to teaching the next generation to be empowered and kind humans who will change the world—starting with her children, Graham and Cambelle.

**Word Search answers from page 38**

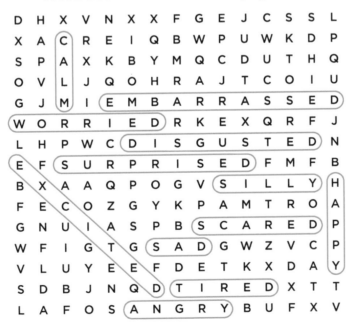

9 781648 766701